It's Time Yoga

Roll Out the Mat

Experience a Yoga Class

BY DIANA DANTUONO, CAS, RYT

Photography by Matthew Siegelbaum

Legwork Team Publishing
New York

AuthorHouse™
1663 Liberty Drive, Suite 200
Bloomington, IN 47403
www.authorhouse.com
Phone: 1-800-839-8640

First published by AuthorHouse 4/7/08

ISBN: 978-1-4343-8257-3 (sc)

Photography by Matthew Siegelbaum
www.strongtreeimages.com

Cover design, interior layout,and print-ready file by the Legwork Team

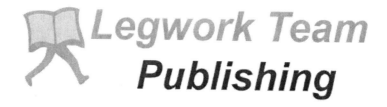

Printed in the United States of America
Bloomington, Indiana

This book is printed on acid-free paper.

This book is dedicated to:
The two most important people in my life,
my parents
John and Grace Dantuono
who have always made my life heaven on earth.

And to
My brothers
Michael and James Dantuono
God's gifts to me.

Contents

Acknowledgments

My main thanks goes to my husband, Pete Cousins, for his time, support, and encouragement throughout this project. Pete, you are special.

I am grateful always to my dear friend Phyllis March who helped in all phases of this project. Her suggestions for and dedication to this book were invaluable.

To Dennis Stallone, whose passion for yoga inspired me to begin my own journey, my profound thanks.

To Grace Welch, Master Yogi, whose knowledge, kindness, compassion, and whose teaching methodologies I try to emulate with my own students, thank you from the bottom of my heart.

It was at the Yoga Teachers Training Institute, Long Island, New York that I deepened my practice and knowledge of yoga principles and, most importantly, learned how to apply these principles to my daily life. I share everything I learned from those instructors with my own students, in hopes that they too will have the same life changing experience that I had. My heartfelt thanks to all of YTTI's teachers and especially to Marianne Mitsinikos, E-RYT, director of asana training; Ma Mokshapriya Shakti, PhD, E-RYT, director of theoretical studies; and Miguel A. Andujar, MD, director of physiological studies.

A special thank you goes to my family and friends for modeling the poses in this book. Pete Cousins; James, Barbara, and Erin Dantuono; and Phyllis and Courtney March: your time and encouragement are very much appreciated.

My appreciation to Rose Zacchi for her support and friendship.

My heartfelt thanks to Ann Mittasch and Lynn Costa for their Feng Shui advice.

I send my appreciation to Yvonne Kamerling, Legwork Team Publishing, who sparked the concept for this book and encouraged me to bring it to fruition.

Introduction

It's Time for Yoga, Roll Out the Mat is invaluable to those seeking a healthier lifestyle. This book offers you the opportunity of attending one of my Hatha yoga classes, a type of yoga that emphasizes physical health, breathing and meditation.

It's Time for Yoga provides you with specific, easy to follow, step by step instruction for each pose. The photographs depict proper body alignment, body posture, and techniques to ensure that even a novice can have a successful and enjoyable yoga experience. The question and answer chapter provides you with a general knowledge of the yogic philosophy, as well as the spiritual, physical, and mental benefits that yoga brings to your life.

Start slowly! You do not have to complete all the postures that are shown in the book during one session. Do as many as you can comfortably. If, at any time, you feel that you need to rest, you may do so. Before ending any yoga session, I recommend that you sit or lie down in a comfortable position and relax for a few minutes.

To compliment this book, I encourage you to seek out a certified yoga instructor who will help you to develop an individualized plan to maximize your yoga practice.

Safety

Check with your health care provider before beginning your yoga practice or any exercise program.

Wear comfortable clothes so your body can breathe and move without constriction.

Practice yoga barefoot so that you are balanced and grounded, and to avoid slipping.

Wait at least one hour after eating before beginning your yoga practice.

Perform postures on a sticky mat or on a nonslip floor so you don't lose your balance.

Modify postures to accommodate special needs. Use props such as bolsters, belts, and blankets for support and comfort. You can also practice some of the postures sitting on a chair or lying in bed. If you have difficulty getting up from the floor, place a chair near your mat. You can use it to support yourself. Skip a posture if you experience any discomfort.

Keep proper head, shoulder, and pelvic alignment to ensure energy flow, prevent injury, and achieve the full benefits of each posture.

Breathe in order to stay calm and focused. Inhale and exhale through your nose. The hairs in your nose clean and warm the air before it enters your body. Never hold your breath.

Do not rush or go beyond your expectations. Progress slowly and at your own pace. Trying to do too much too quickly may cause injury. Listen to your body. Everyone is different. Use common sense. Put your ego and pride aside.

Have patience. You may never achieve a certain posture or it may take some time. Take it day-by-day. Some days are better than others.

Rest in Corpse Pose, illustrated on page 82, after you have done several postures. It allows you to rest, and it also gives your body a chance to remember the postures.

Hello!

My name is Diana. Welcome to my yoga class.
I am your yoga instructor. I would like to introduce you to the students pictured in this book. They represent a typical yoga class composed of various levels of ability.

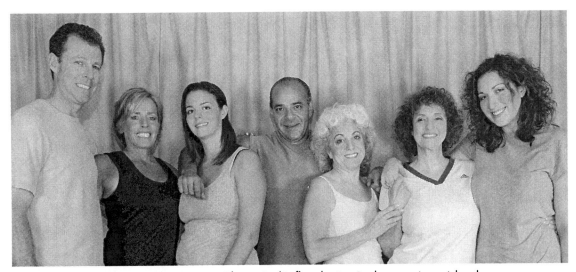

FROM LEFT TO RIGHT: Pete, Massage Therapist/Reflexologist; Barbara, a Long Island, NY School District Employee; Erin, Physical Therapy Student; Jim, Nassau County, New York, Department of Corrections, Diana, Your Yoga Instructor, Phyllis, Special Education Teacher; and Courtney, Psychology Student.

This lesson will begin with a deep breathing exercise followed by the yoga asanas (postures). We will conclude with relaxation and meditation.

Remember To:
Stop if experiencing any pain or discomfort.
Breathe slowly and deeply throughout the practice.
Experience the joy.

So...IT'S TIME FOR YOGA, ROLL OUT THE MAT
Let's begin the journey together.

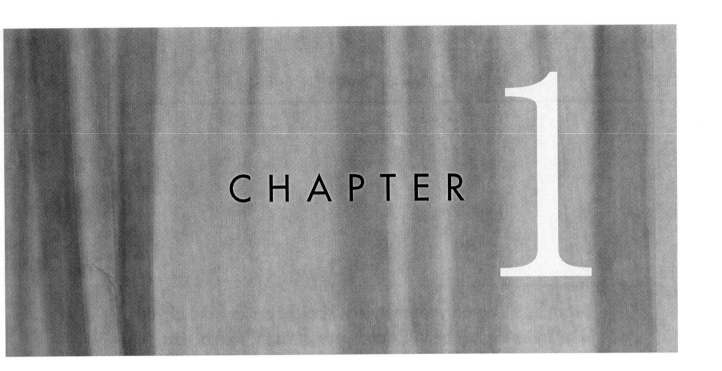

CHAPTER 1

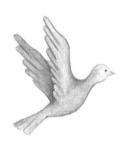

Breathing

Begin by sitting on your mat, legs straight out in front of you with knees slightly bent. Extend your arms in front of you, interlock your thumbs, tighten your stomach, and slowly begin to ease down vertebra by vertebra until you are resting on your back.

Place hands below the navel, fingers touching, and focus your attention on your breath. Breathe naturally.

Now, begin to slow down your breathing, inhaling and exhaling through your nose. As you inhale your stomach rises, fingers part and as you exhale your stomach falls, fingers touch. Your breathing should be slow, deep, and with rhythm. Just like an ocean wave, as you inhale stomach rises the wave goes to the shore. Exhale stomach falls, the wave returns to the ocean. Focus on your breath. Breathe for a few minutes.

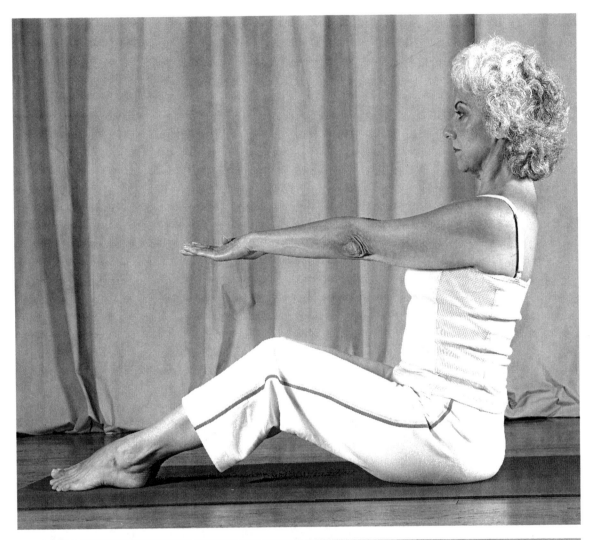

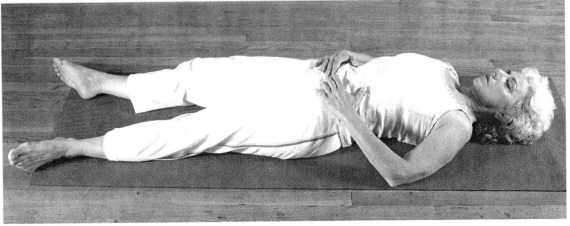

CHAPTER 2

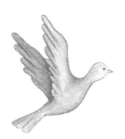

Supine Poses
and
Stretches

While lying on your back, bring your legs together, arms overhead, touching the floor, point your toes, take a deep breath, and stretch giving space between each vertebra.

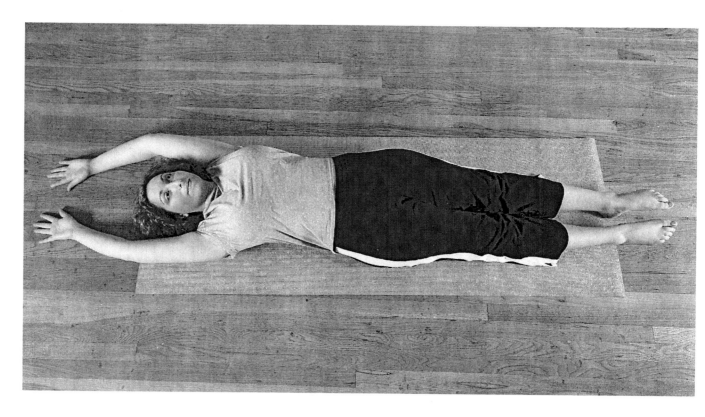

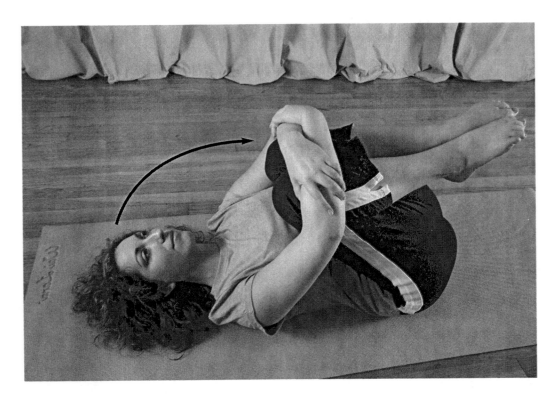

Knee Hug Pose

This asana stretches the lower back muscles while massaging the entire back.

Bring your knees to your chest and hug them. Inhale. As you exhale bring your head and chest up to meet your knees. Take slow, deep breaths.

To prepare for Windshield Wiper, bring your head, chest, and feet down to the floor keeping your knees bent and your feet hip width apart. Stretch your arms out to the side, level with your shoulders, in T position.

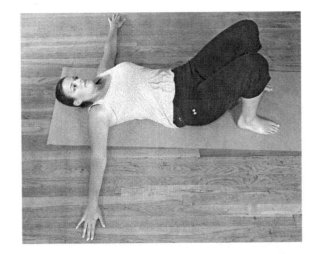

Windshield Wiper Pose

This movement relieves headaches and cleanses the digestive system.

Inhale. As you exhale drop your knees to the right and turn your head to the left.

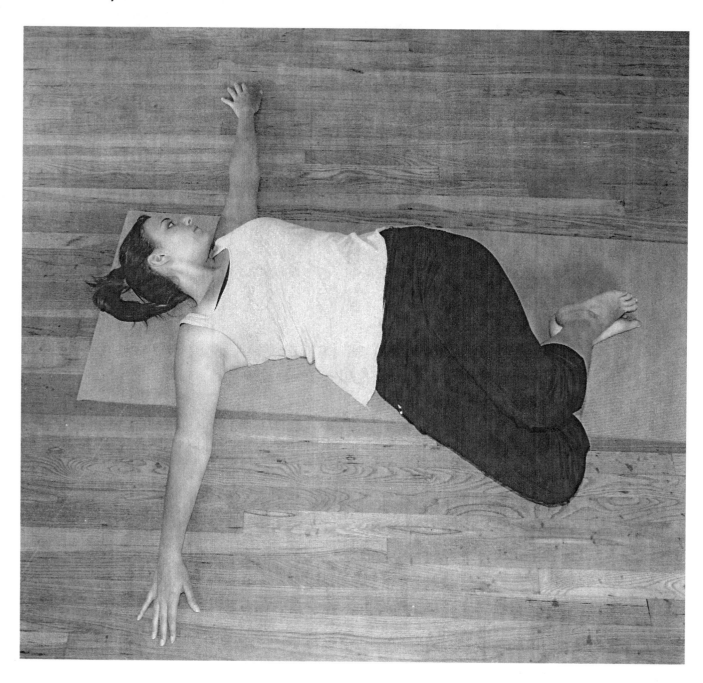

Inhale. Exhale, dropping your knees to the left and turning your head to the right. Continue this several times and then return to center.

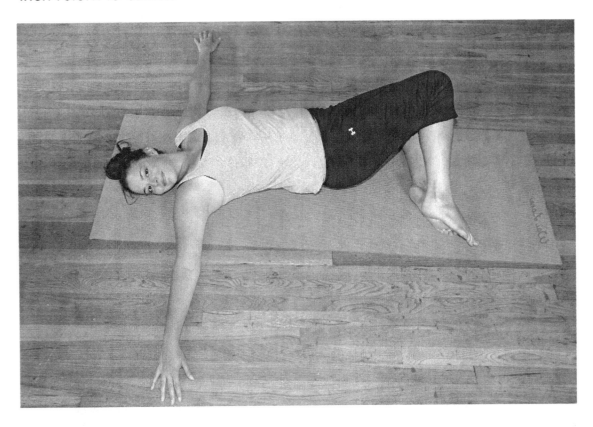

Bring your knees to your chest and hug them as you press your lower back to the floor.

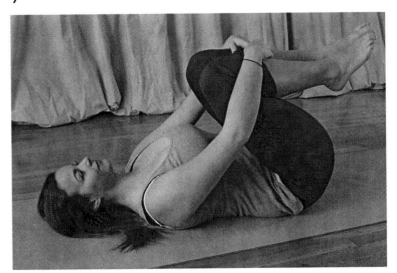

Happy Baby Pose

This pose releases the lower back, opens hips, inner thighs, and groin.

Place your arms between your knees, lift your head and chest, hold the outer edges of the feet, and then rest your head and chest back on the floor. Stay in this position for three breaths.

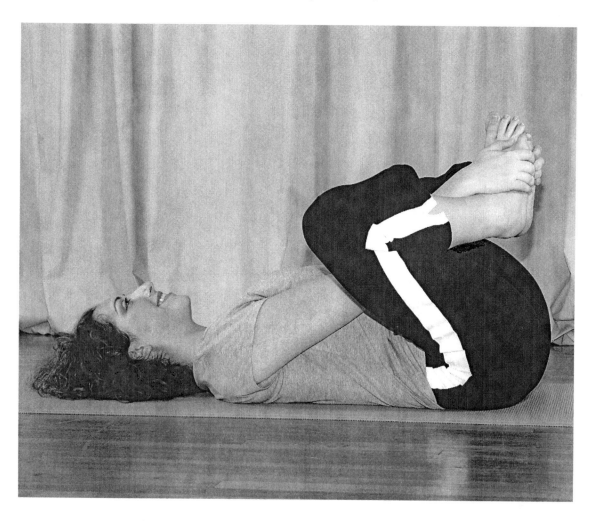

Yoga Toe Lock Pose

Wrap the thumb and first two fingers of your left hand around your left big toe; do the same with your right hand and toe.

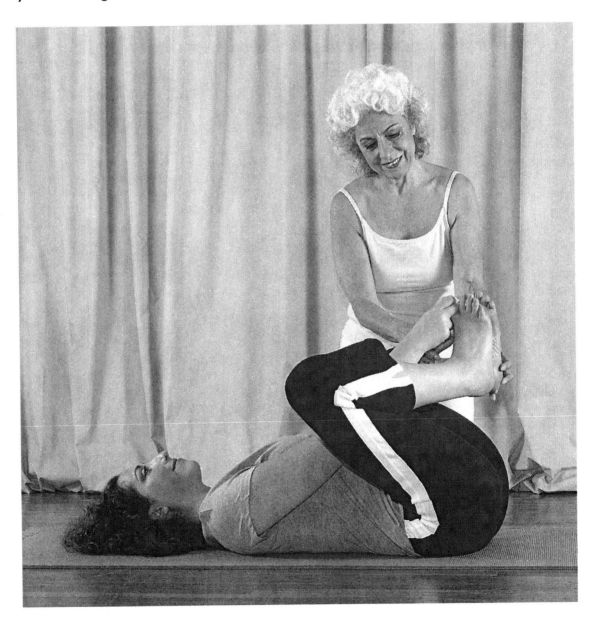

Legs to Ceiling Pose
This relaxes leg muscles and enhances the circulatory system.

Extend your legs to the ceiling as you press your tailbone
down to the floor. Relax your shoulders. Continue to breathe.
If your legs won't straighten, bend them slightly.

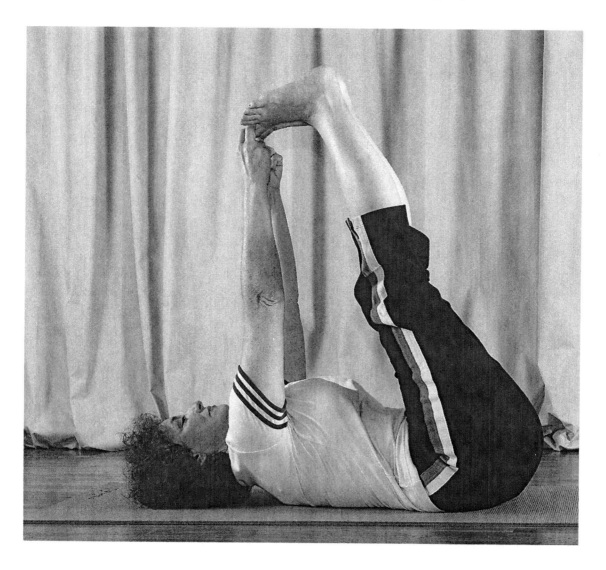

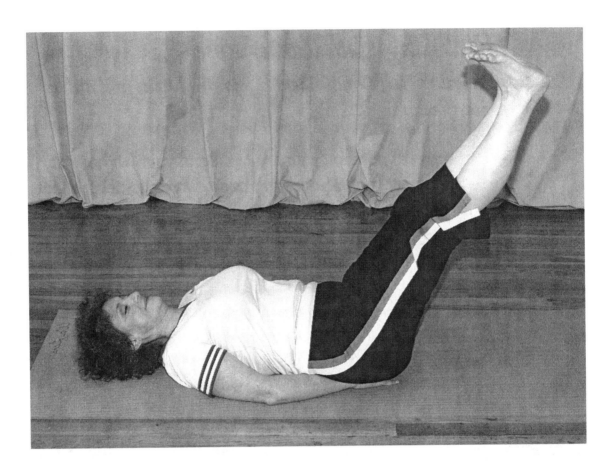

Release Yoga Toe Lock
This tones the stomach.

After releasing your toes, place your hands under your buttocks to protect your back, flex your feet, tighten your stomach, and on a slow count of ten, bring your legs down to the floor (ten—nine—eight—seven—six—five—four—three—two—one).

Release your arms from underneath your buttocks.

Reclining Half Lotus Pose

Reclining Half Lotus makes hip joints, knees, and ankles more flexible.

Place your left hand on your left hip. Bend your left knee as you bring your foot to your right hand, which guides the foot to rest on the right thigh. Allow your knee to drop to the side. The right leg is active by keeping the foot flexed. Stay in this position for three breaths.

Release and bring the leg down to the floor.

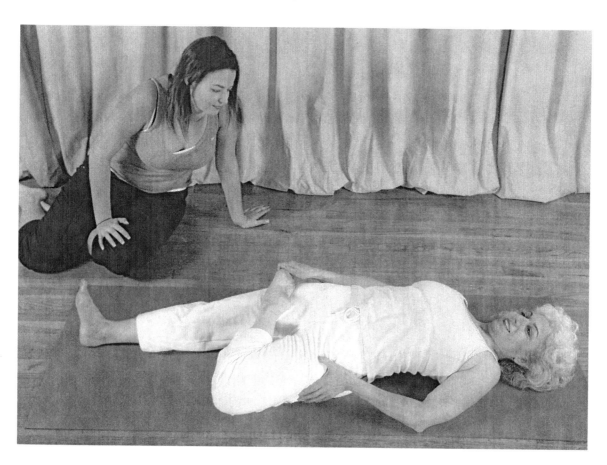

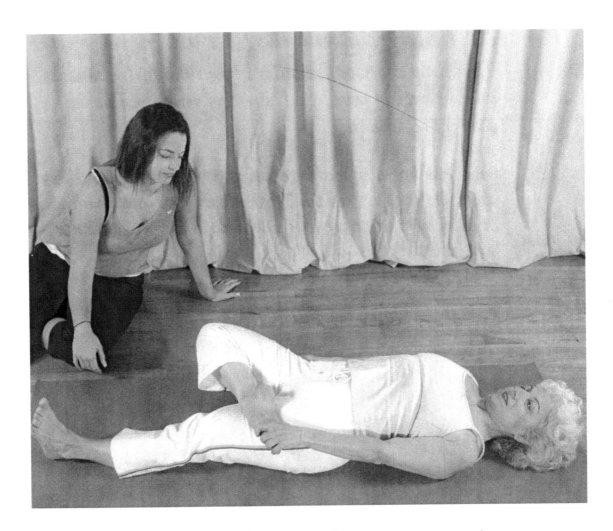

Repeat on the other side. Place your right hand on your right hip. Bend the right knee and bring the right foot to the left hand, which guides the foot to rest on the left thigh. Allow the knee to drop to the side. The left leg is active and the foot flexed. Take three deep breaths.

Reclining Bound Angle Pose

This asana develops flexibility in your hamstring muscles and the back of your legs. It stretches your groin and is good for relaxation.

Bend your knees so that the soles of your feet touch and your knees drop out to the side. Either stretch your arms overhead or relax them down by your side. Rest in this position for three breaths.

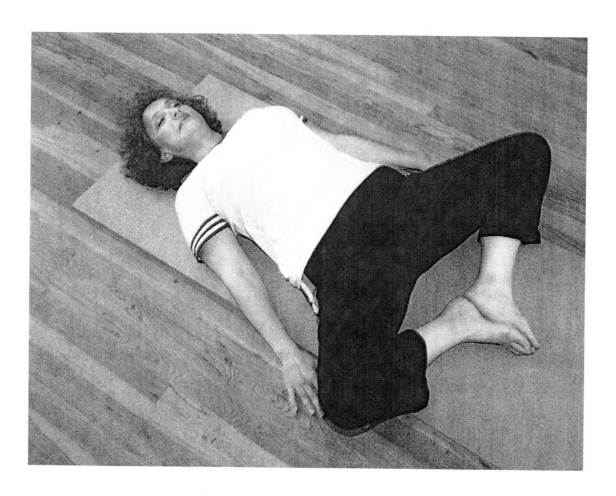

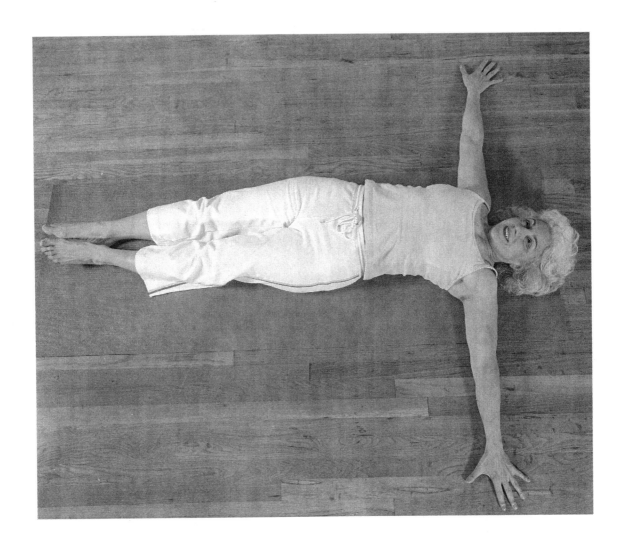

Supine Revolved Triangle Pose

Supine Revolved Triangle strengthens and stretches the hips and spine, and relieves mild back pain.

Straighten out your legs. Place your arms palms down, in line with your shoulders in T position.

Raise your right leg and slowly move it across your body to the left and rest the foot on the floor.

Relax your shoulders and turn your head to the right. Breathe.

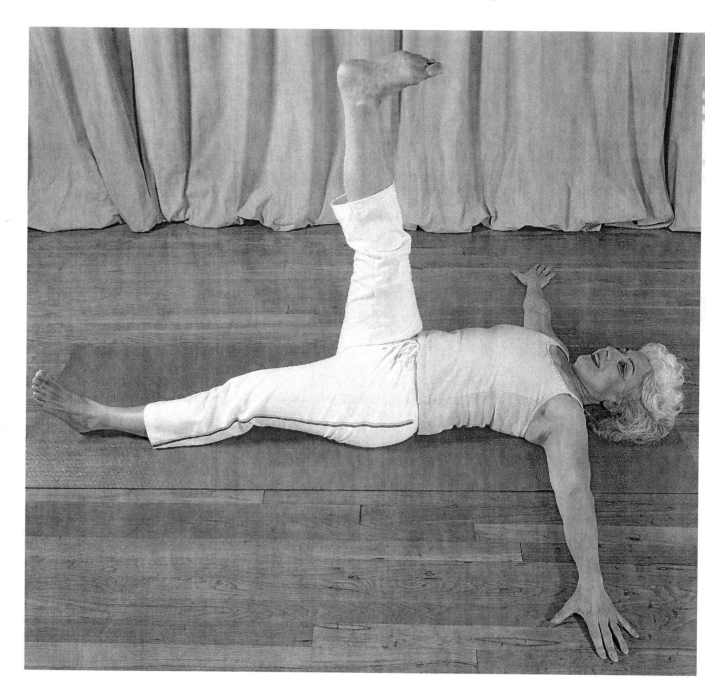

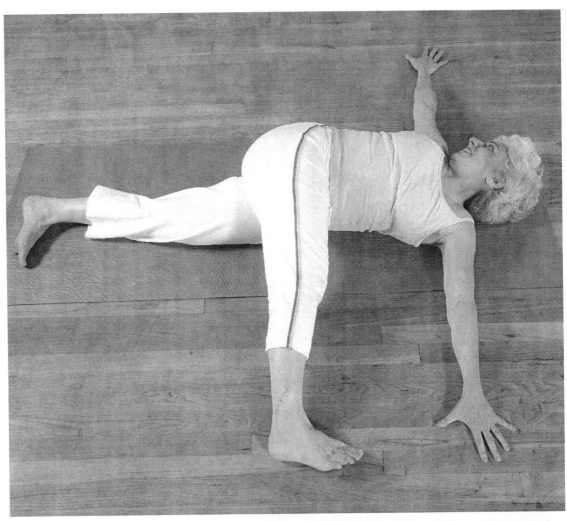

Lift the right leg to the ceiling
and back down to the floor.

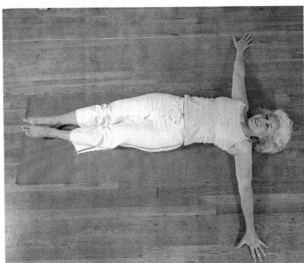

Repeat on the other side. Raise your left leg and slowly move it across your body to the right and rest the foot on the floor.

Relax your shoulders and turn your head to the left. Don't forget to breathe.

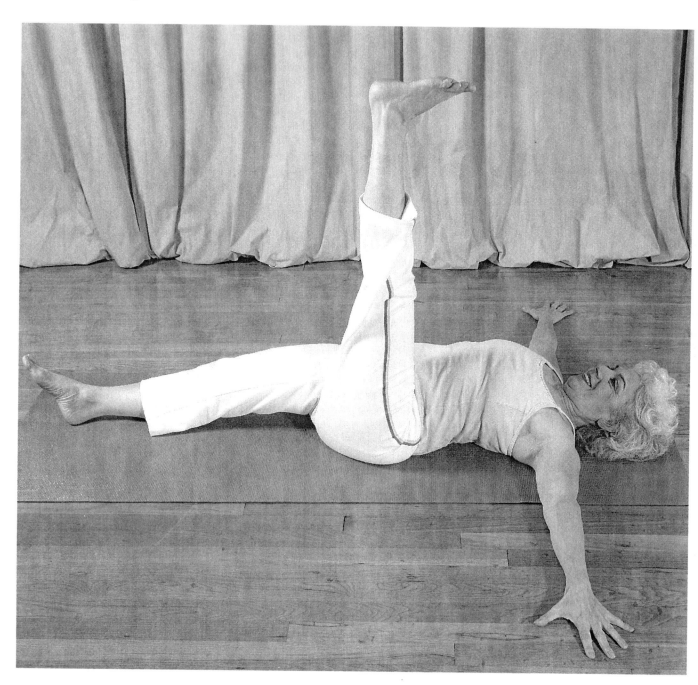

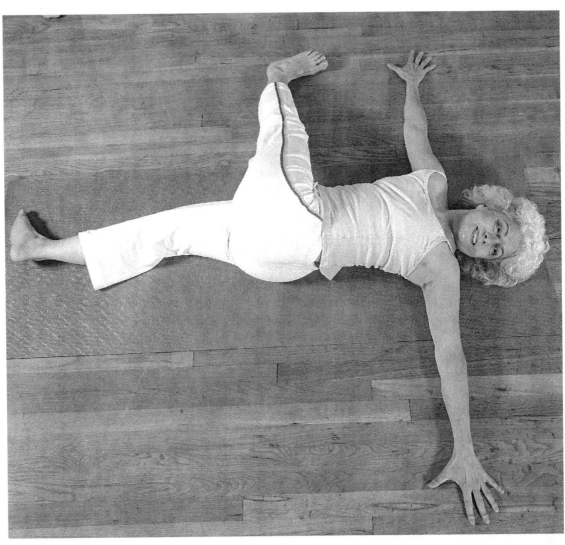

Lift the left leg to the ceiling and back down to the floor.

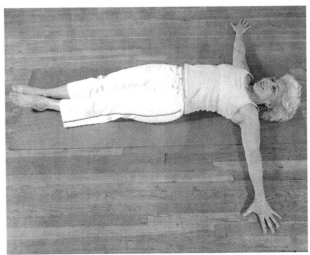

CHAPTER 3

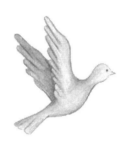

Seated Poses
and
Stretches

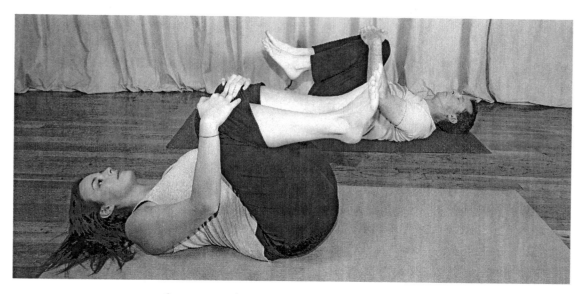

Prepare for seated position.

Bring your legs together, bend your knees to your chest and roll to the right into a fetal position.

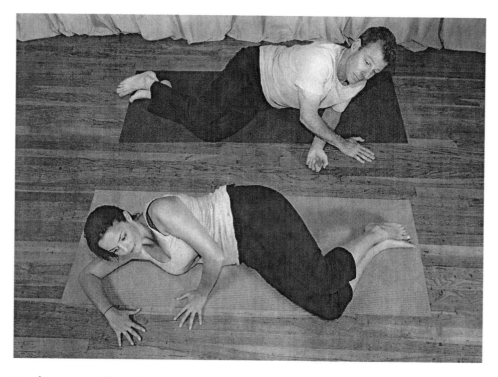

Push yourself up by using your arms and not your back.

Bound Angle Pose

Bound Angle stretches inner thighs, groin, and knees.
It soothes menstrual discomfort and sciatica. If you have
a knee injury, it's advised that you don't do this pose.

Sit with your legs stretched out in front of you.

Bend the knees and pull the feet toward the groin. Let the knees fall to the side and the soles of the feet touch. Hold your toes or your ankles. Sit up tall. Relax your shoulders and breathe.

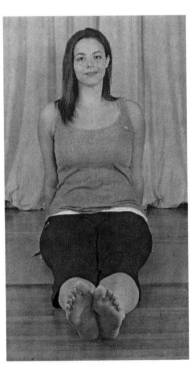

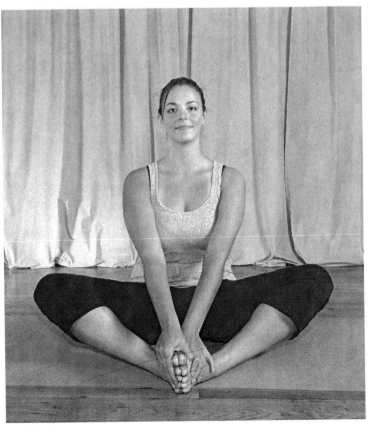

ON THE BLACKBOARD

While in a seated position, notice if you are slouching. If so, lift your chest. This will ensure an erect posture.

Staff Pose

Staff Pose improves posture and strengthens the back muscles.

Lift your knees away from the floor and extend your legs out
in front of you. Rest your hands by your side or on your
thighs. Breathe.

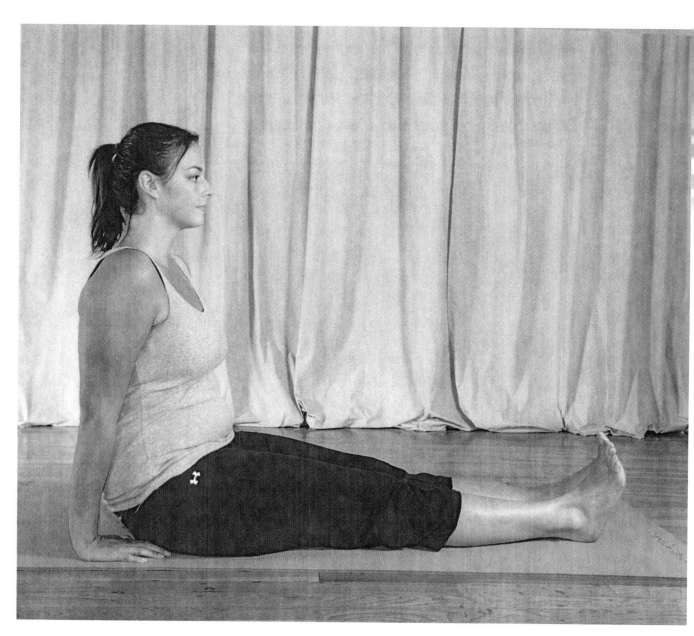

Cross-Legged Seated Pose
This stretches the back and inner thighs.

Sit with your legs crossed. Allow your knees to lower.
Place your hands on your knees; sit up tall.

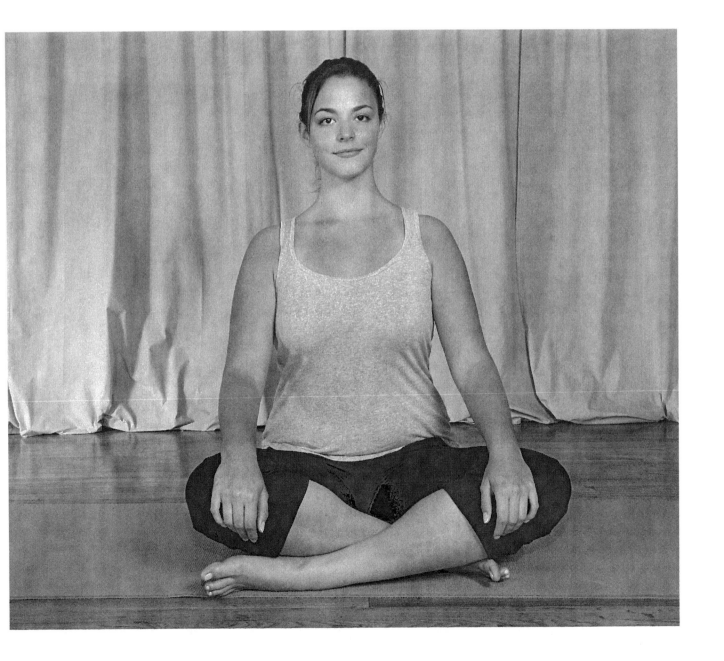

Neck and Shoulder Stretches

This relaxes the head and face, and stretches the neck. The stretches promote flexibility and range of motion, and offer relief for tight shoulders.

Begin by relaxing your chin to your chest and then allow your head to gently fall back. Continue breathing as you flow from chin to chest and head back.

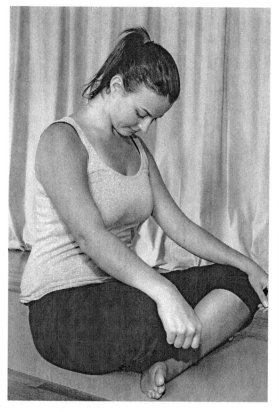 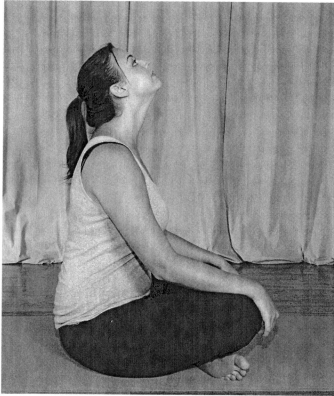

Return to center.

Slowly look to your left. Look to your right. Continue breathing slowly as you look from one side to the other.

Return to center.

Bring your right ear to your shoulder and stretch your left shoulder down away from your ear.

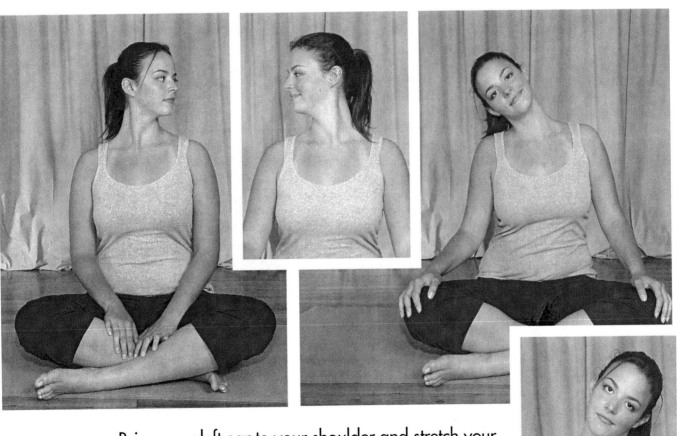

Bring your left ear to your shoulder and stretch your right shoulder down away from your ear. Continue several times while breathing.

Return to center.

Make three big circles with your shoulders, first going forward and then going back.

Return to center.

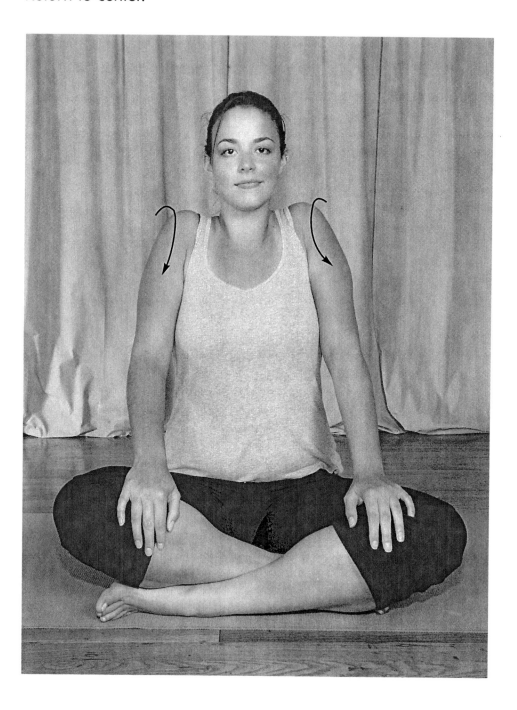

Place your hands on your shoulders and slowly make three big circles with your elbows each way.

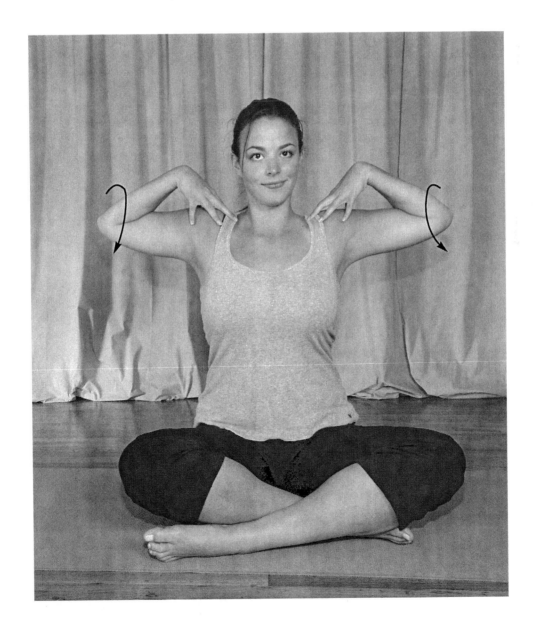

Stretch your arms out in front of you, palms facing out. Cross your right arm over left so that your palms touch. Breathe softly.

Now, reverse left arm over right.

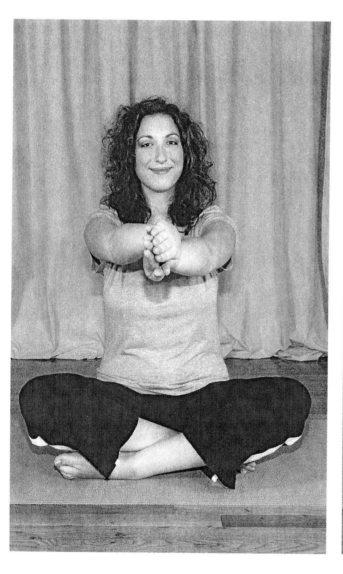 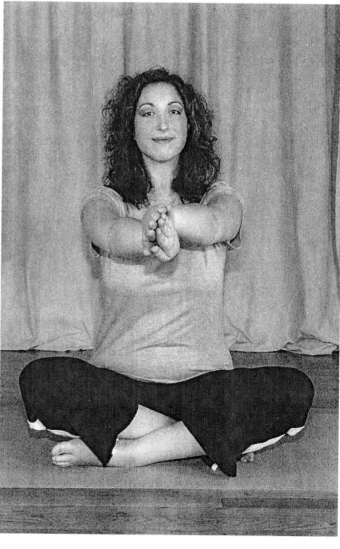

Clasp your hands and flip, palms are now facing out. Stretch your wrists, palms, and fingers.

Lift arms overhead and then release your hands. With palms facing in, bring your arms down by your side. Move slowly as if energy is pulling them down.

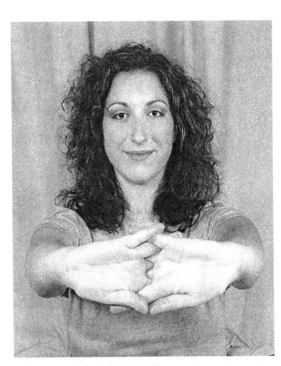

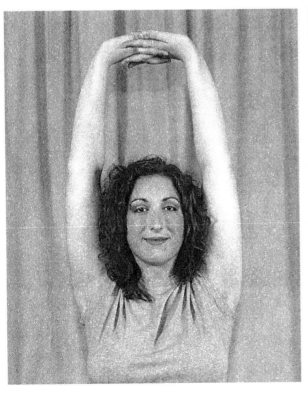

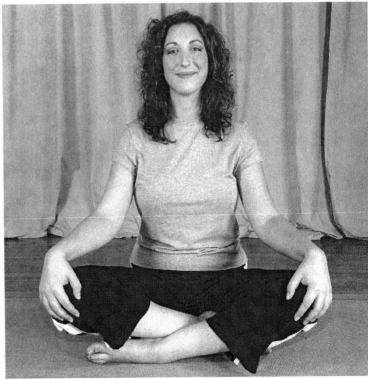

The next stretch is to bring your arms behind you, clasp your hands, roll your shoulders back, and slowly lift your arms to where it is comfortable—you may have to loosen the grip. Take three breaths.

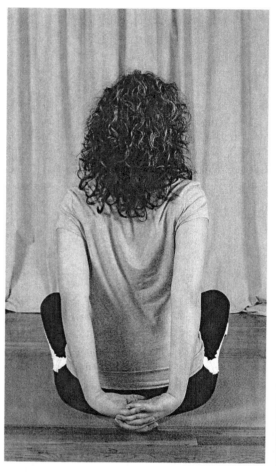
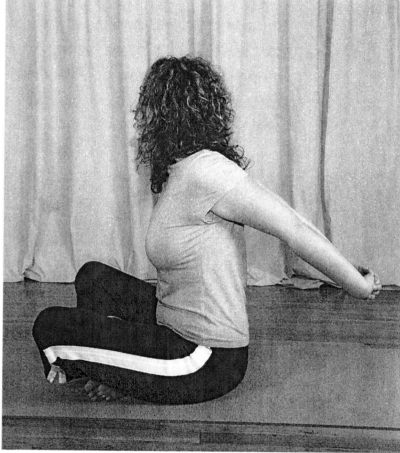

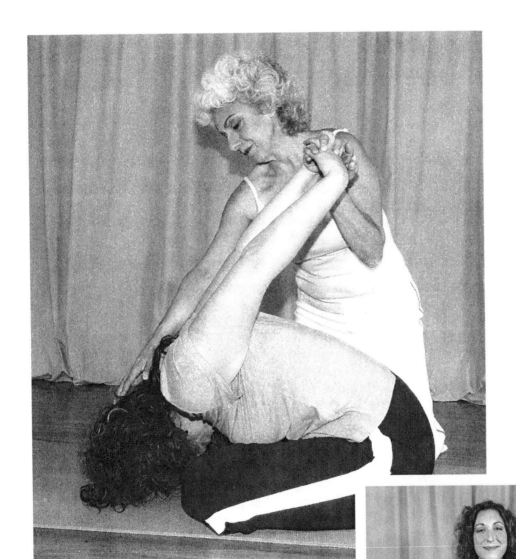

On your last exhale, bend forward, continuing to lift your arms. Relax in this position for a moment.

On an exhale slowly return to a seated position and release your arms.

Side Stretch

This stretch increases flexibility of your spine, arms, and rib cage.

Place your right hand on your left knee. As you inhale your left arm goes up. As you exhale stretch your arm overhead and to the right.

Hold for a few breaths. Inhale. Stretch your left arm up. Exhale. Bring your left arm down to your side.

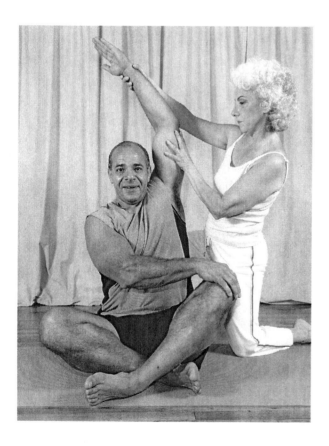
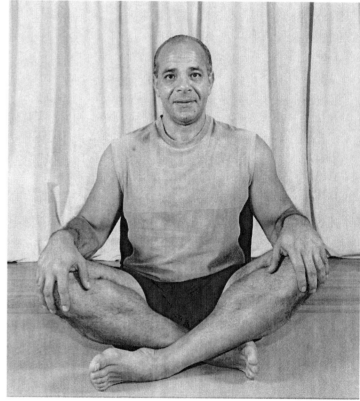

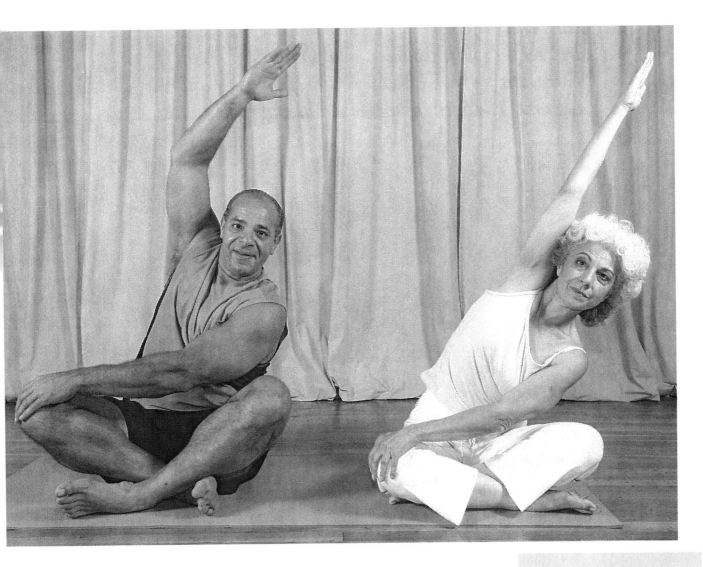

Repeat with the left hand. Place your left hand on your right knee. As you inhale your right arm goes up. As you exhale stretch your arm overhead and to the left. Hold for a few breaths. Inhale. Stretch your right arm up. Exhale. Bring your right arm down to your side.

ON THE BLACKBOARD

Many seated postures can be done on a chair, while at work, on an airplane, or watching TV.

Seated Forward Bend Pose

This bend helps relieve stress and mild depression. It stretches the spine, shoulders, and hamstrings and is therapeutic for high blood pressure. If you have asthma, diarrhea, or a back injury, do not attempt this asana.

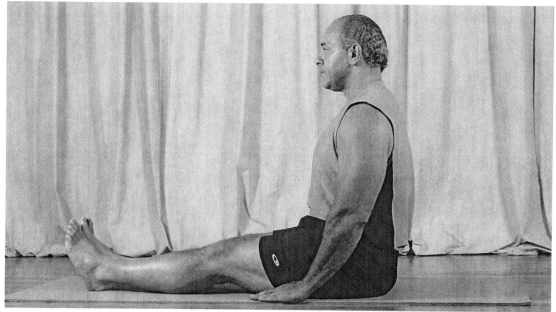

Straighten your legs out in front of you, arms by your side.

As you inhale lift your arms out to the side and stretch up.

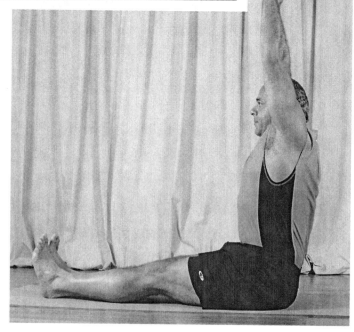

Exhale, bending forward. Lead with your chin and chest to elongate your spine. Hold onto your shinbones, ankles, or feet.

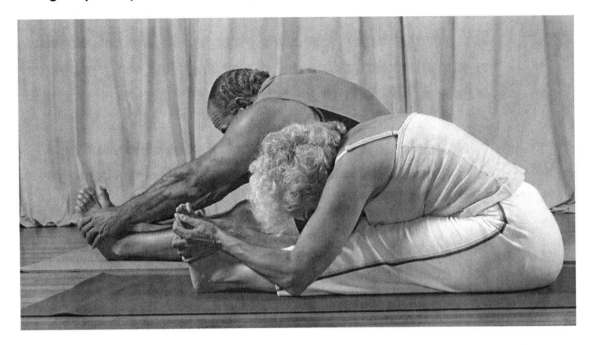

Move your tailbone back so your chest touches your thighs. Part your legs if your stomach is in the way. Remain here for three breaths.

Bring your hands together, inhale, and lift your arms overhead.

Exhale, arms down by your side.

ON THE BLACKBOARD

While doing the postures, do not hold your breath as this can raise your blood pressure.

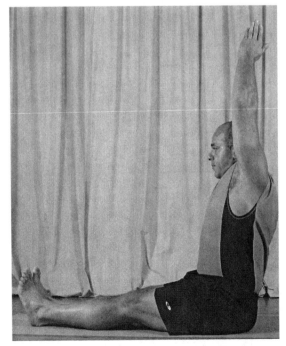

Head to Knee Pose

As with Seated Forward Bend, Head to Knee Pose stretches the spine, shoulders, and hamstrings, as well as the groin. It is therapeutic for high blood pressure and also for insomnia. If you are experiencing asthma or diarrhea, or if you have a knee injury, do not try this pose.

Sit with your legs extended in front of you. Bend your right leg and bring the foot close to the groin—this will bring your knee to the floor.

Tilt your tailbone back so that you are sitting upright—keep your back straight.

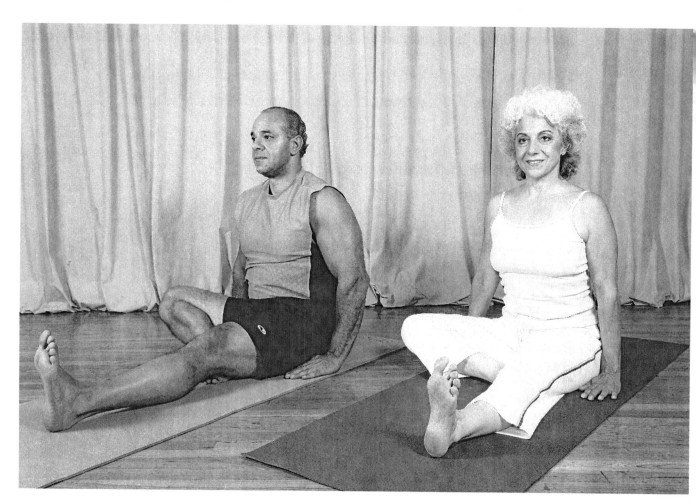

Inhale, lifting your arms out and up.

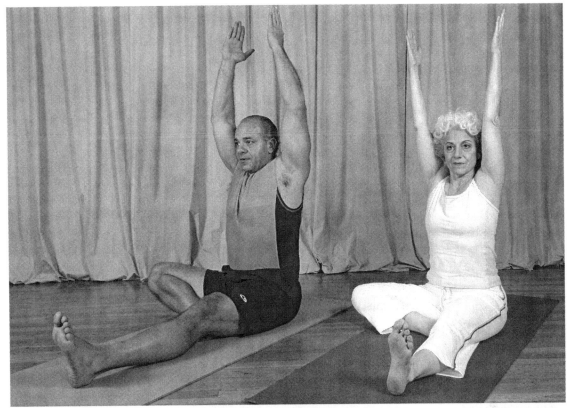

Exhale, bending forward. Lead with your chin and chest. Hold for three breaths.

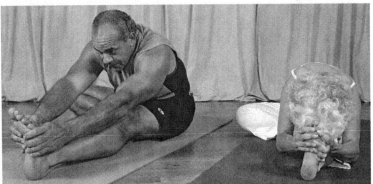

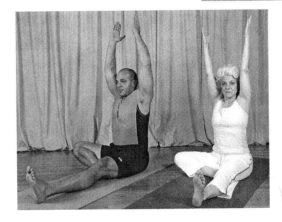

Coming out of Head to Knee Pose.
Bring your hands together, inhale, and lift your arms overhead. Exhale, and rest your arms down by your side.

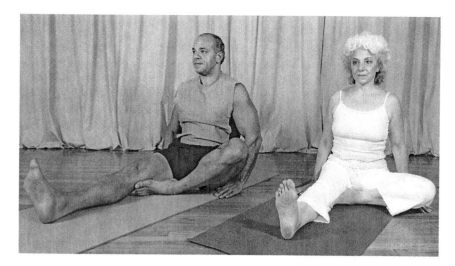

Repeat Head to Knee for your left side.

Bring your hands together, inhale, and lift your arms overhead.

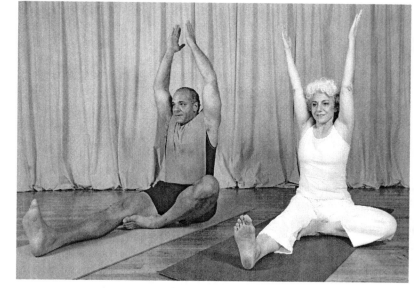

Exhale, bending forward. Lead with your chin and chest. Hold for three breaths.

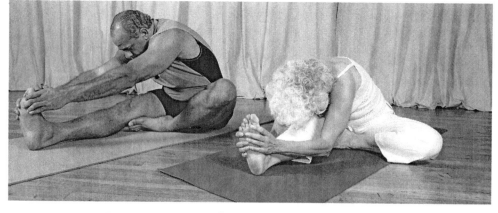

Coming out of Head to Knee Pose.
Bring your hands together, inhale, and lift your arms overhead. Exhale, and rest your arms down by your side.

CHAPTER 4

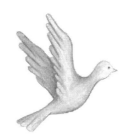

Floor Poses

Table Pose

Move onto all fours for Table. Make sure your wrists are under your shoulders, your knees are under your hips, and your fingers are spread wide with the middle fingers pointed straight ahead.

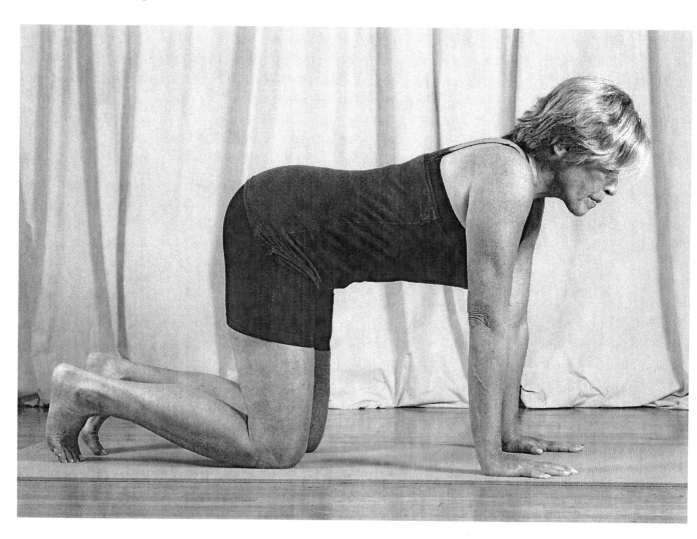

Cow and Cat Pose

Cow and Cat Pose increases flexibility of the spine, improves circulation, and stretches muscles along the neck, back, and arms.

Curl your toes under. For Cow, inhale and lift your head and tailbone. This curls your spine downward. Exhale and relax your head and tailbone down. This arches your back, forming Cat.

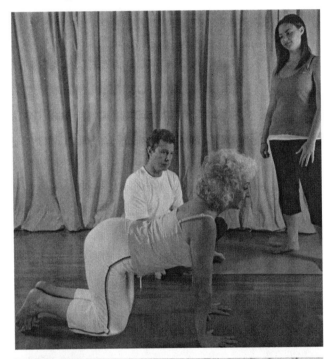

Repeat several times, flowing from Cow to Cat, Cat to Cow. Inhale and exhale as you slowly move into each pose.

Return to Table, remembering to place your hands under your shoulders and your knees under your hips. Spread your fingers wide, the middle fingers pointed straight ahead.

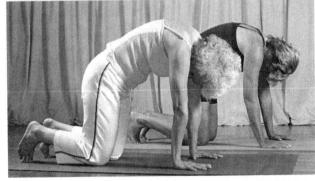

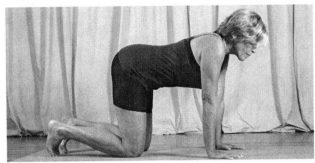

Downward Facing Dog Pose

This aligns and strengthens the spine; releases tension in the shoulders; strengthens and stretches the hamstrings, hands, wrists, arms, and shoulders; and helps prevent shoulders from rounding forward.

Curl your toes under. Glide your tailbone back as you lift your hips and straighten your legs. Keep your feet hip width apart. Press your feet and hands firmly onto the floor. Relax your head and neck. Gaze at your navel. Take three slow, deep breaths.

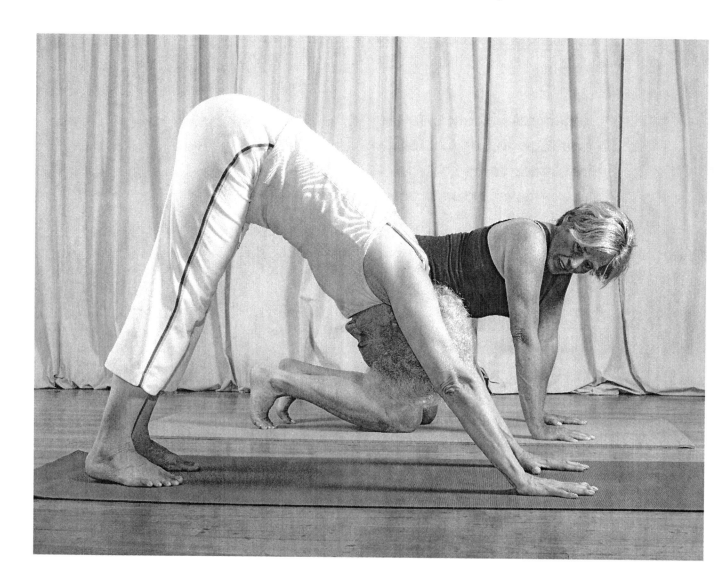

Child's Pose

Resting in Child's Pose stretches hips, thighs, and ankles. It helps relieve stress and fatigue, and it massages the inner organs. If you have diarrhea or are pregnant, it's advised that you don't sit in this pose. If you have a knee injury, or if the pose causes discomfort to your knee, place a folded blanket or towel in the fold of your knee or under your toes.

Bring your knees down, uncurl your toes, and come into Child's Pose by sitting back on your heels with your forehead down and your arms by your sides, palms up. Remember to breathe. If this pose is uncomfortable, rest on your side.

Come up to standing on your knees.

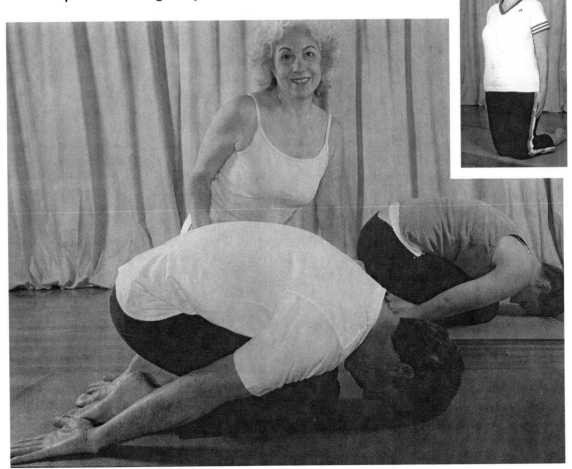

Gate Pose

Gate Pose stretches the sides of the torso, as well as the spine and hamstrings. Do not attempt this asana if you have a knee injury.

Extend your right leg out to the right side. Make sure your left knee is in line with your left hip. Arms by your side. On an exhale stretch your left arm up and to the side. Continue to breathe.

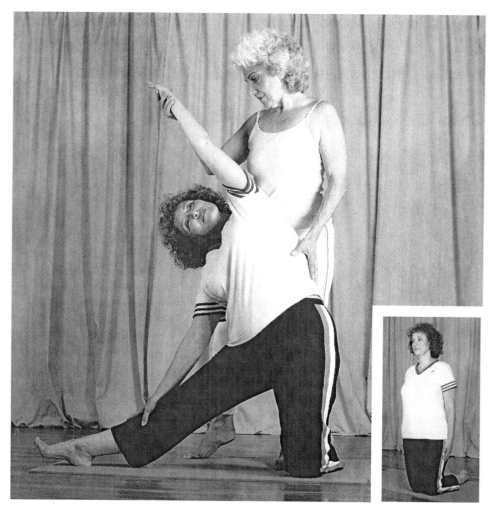

To come out of this pose, inhale your left arm up and exhale the arm down by your side. Bring knees together.

Repeat Gate Pose on the other side. Extend your left leg out to the left side. Make sure your right knee is in line with your right hip. Arms by your side. On an exhale stretch your right arm up and to the side. Continue to breathe.

To come out of this pose, inhale your right arm up and exhale the arm down by your side.

Bring knees together.

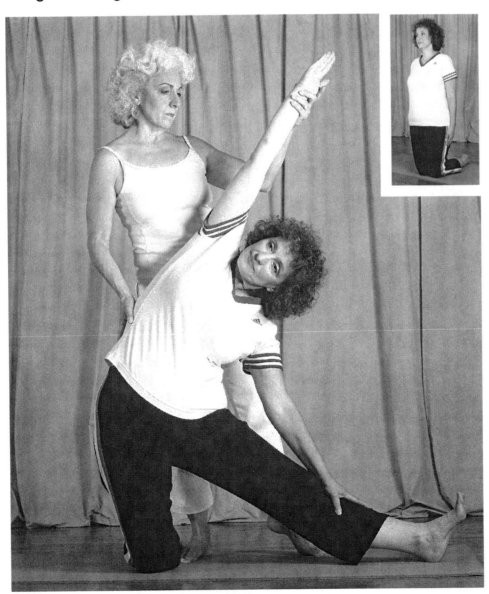

CHAPTER 5

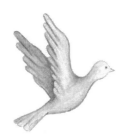

Prone Poses

Slowly lie on your stomach and stretch your arms overhead, taking deep breaths.

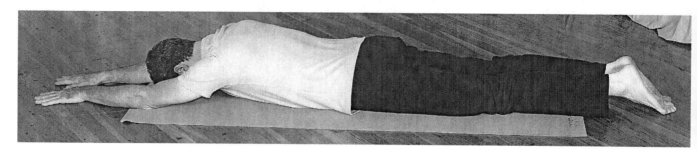

Cobra Pose

This strengthens the spine; stretches the chest, shoulders, and abdomen; firms the buttocks; and soothes sciatica. Back injury, carpal tunnel syndrome, or pregnancy may prevent you from completing this position.

Place your hands under your shoulders, fingers spread wide, elbows close to your body. Point your forehead down. Inhale and glide your forehead, nose, and chin. Exhale and lift your head and chest up, keeping your hips down, and tighten your buttocks. Continue to breathe.

On an exhale slowly lower yourself down.

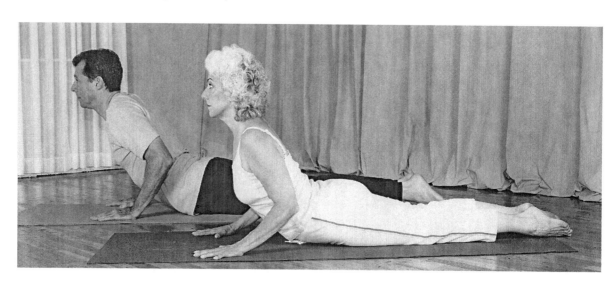

Upward Facing Dog Pose

Up Dog strengthens the spine, arms, and wrists. It stretches the chest, shoulders, and abdomen; firms the buttocks; and helps relieve sciatica. As with Cobra Pose, you should not try Upward Facing Dog if you have a back injury or carpal tunnel syndrome, or if you are pregnant.

Walk your hands down just a few inches, fingers spread wide. Inhale, as you exhale head, chest and hips come up, arms are straight. Take three breaths.

Exhale come down onto your stomach.

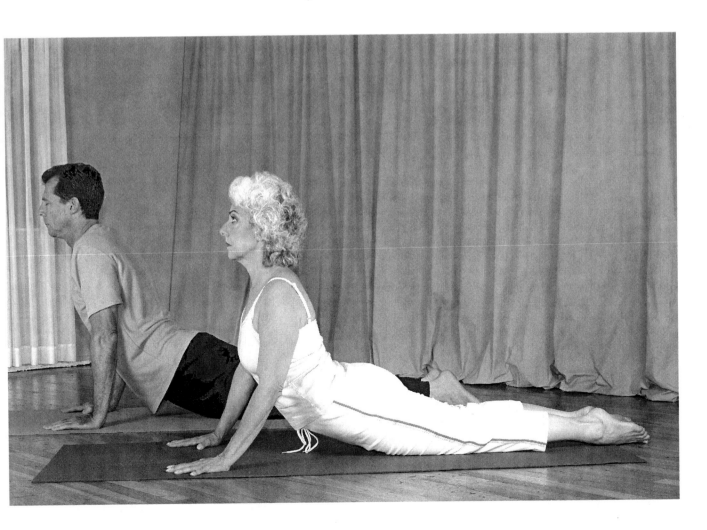

CHAPTER 6

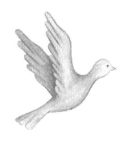

Standing Poses

Now slowly come to a standing position.

Mountain Pose

This improves posture and balance, relieves sciatica, firms the abdomen and buttocks, and strengthens the thighs, knees, and ankles.

Touch your big toes together; all other toes are separated. Lift your right heel, stretching the sole of your foot. Lower your right heel and lift your left heel. Lower it. Drop your shoulders away and slightly back from your ears. Chin parallel to the floor, glide your head back just a little so that your ears, shoulders, and hips are in alignment. Tuck your tailbone under. Relax your arms by your side.

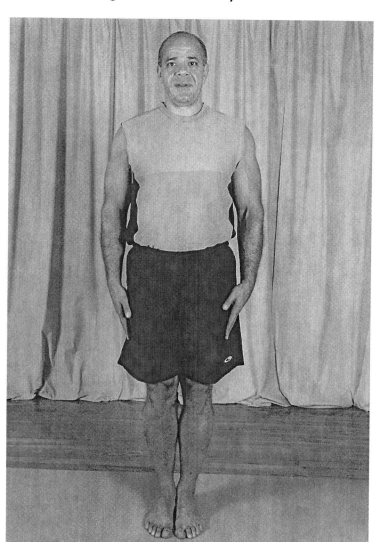

ON THE BLACKBOARD

Standing poses gives you the opportunity to envision yourself as physically, mentally, and spiritually strong.

Chair Pose

It strengthens the ankles, thighs, calves, and spine. It stretches the shoulders and chest. If your heels ache or you have insomnia, do not try this position.

Stand as you did for Mountain Pose, your big toes touching. Inhale, arms out to the side and up; palms touch. Exhale, bend your knees, and pretend you are sitting on a chair by extending your tailbone out. Arms, head, and chest stretch up and back. Breathe.

Coming out of Chair

Bring your head back to center and stand up straight. Place your arms down by your side.

Tree Pose

Tree develops concentration, balance, coordination, and strength.

Shift your weight to your left foot and firm that leg. Bend your right leg, lifting the foot off the floor and placing the foot as high as possible against your left inner thigh. Make sure the knee is out to the side. Press your palms together in prayer in front of your heart or your palms together over your head. Focus on a point at eye level in the distance. If you feel unstable, lower your foot to the calf or ankle. Keep focusing and breathing.

To come out of Tree, bring your arms down by your side and release your foot to the floor.

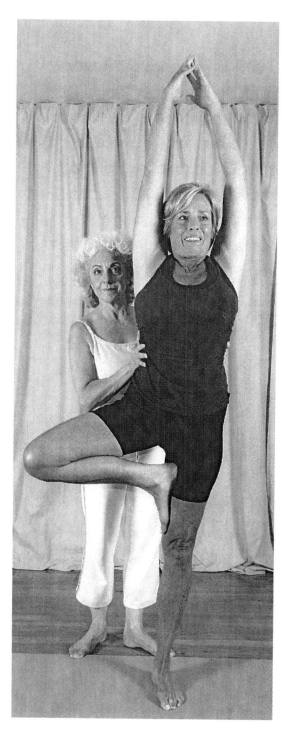

Now, shift your weight to your right foot and firm that leg. Bend your left leg, lifting the foot off the floor and placing the foot as high as possible against your right inner thigh. Make sure the knee is out to the side. Press your palms together in prayer in front of your heart or your palms together over your head. Focus on a point at eye level in the distance. If you feel unstable, lower your foot to the calf or ankle. Keep focusing and breathing.

To come out of Tree, arms down by your side, and release the foot to the floor.

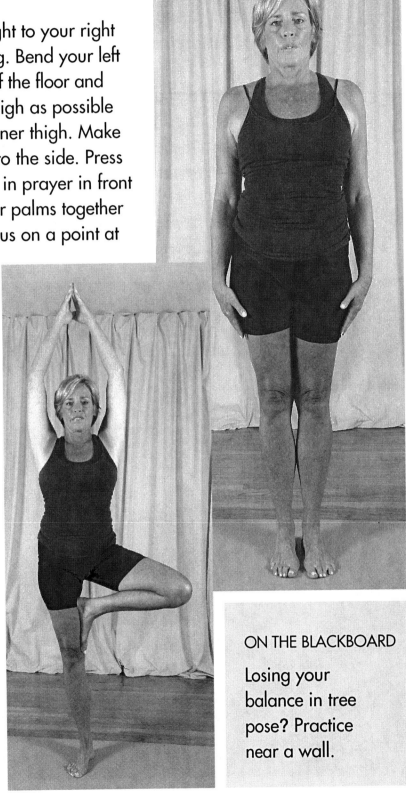

ON THE BLACKBOARD

Losing your balance in tree pose? Practice near a wall.

Triangle Pose

Triangle strengthens the ankles and tones leg muscles. This pose is not recommended for people with hamstring injuries.

Place your right leg at 90 degrees. That's placing your foot out to the side. Legs are three or four feet apart, heel to instep alignment. Turn the left leg slightly to the left, square your hips forward. On an exhale bring your arms in T position. Stretch your left hip out, and right arm stretching forward, tuck your tailbone under. Place your right hand on to your leg, left hand on your waist, turn your chest and head forward and up.

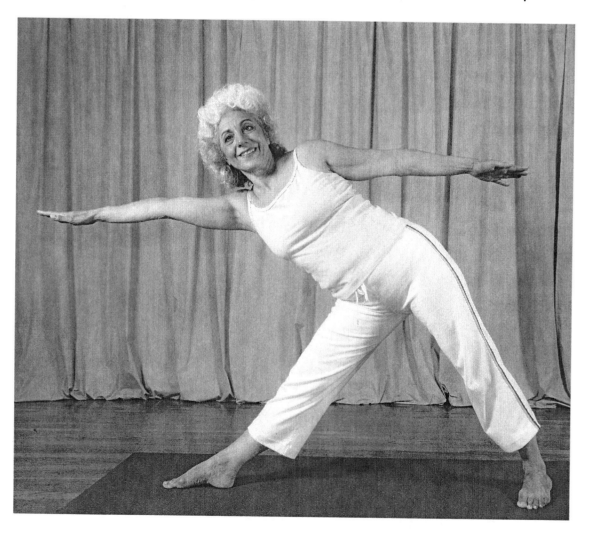

Stretch your left arm to the ceiling. Relax your shoulders and gaze at your finger tips. Stay here for three breaths.

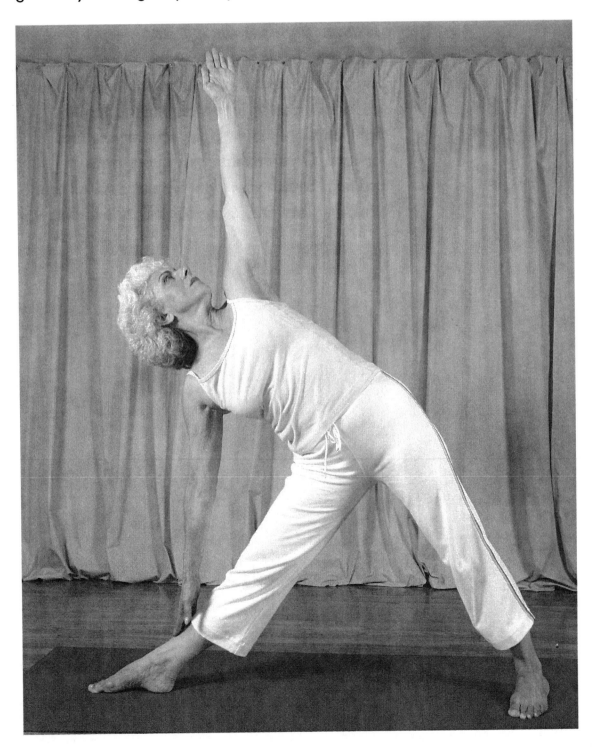

To come out of Triangle Pose
On the exhale bring your arm down and come to standing position, toes pointed forward and step your feet together.

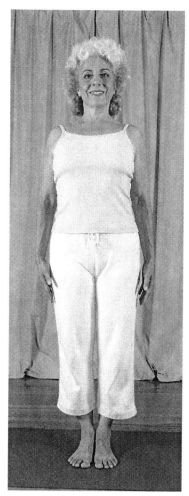

Triangle Pose on the left side
Place your left leg at 90 degrees. That's placing your foot out to the side. Legs are three or four feet apart, heel to instep alignment. Turn the right leg slightly to the right, square your hips forward. On an exhale bring your arms in T position. Stretch your right hip out, and left arm stretching forward, tuck your tailbone under.

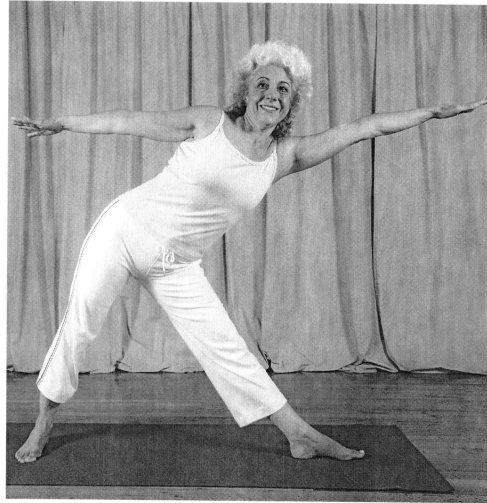

Place your left hand on to your leg, right hand on your waist, turn your chest and head forward and up.

Stretch your right arm to the ceiling. Relax your shoulders and gaze at your finger tips. Stay here for three breaths.

To come out of Triangle Pose
On the exhale bring your arm down and come to standing position, toes pointed forward and step your feet together.

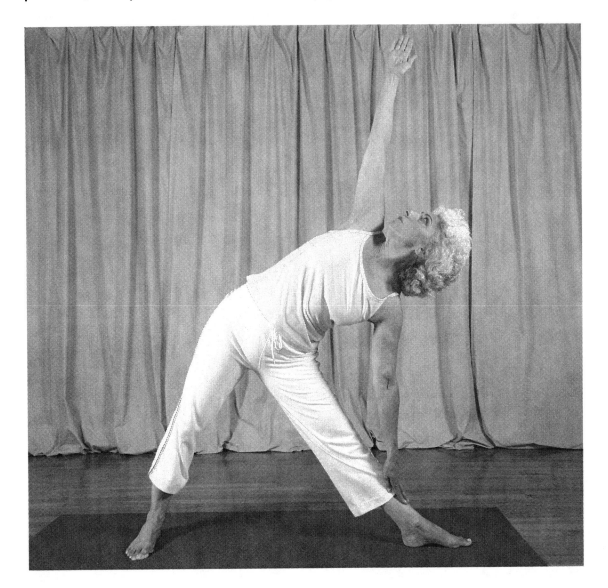

Warrior II Pose

This pose strengthens the legs, arms, and ankles; stretches the groin, chest, and shoulders; increases stamina; and improves balance and coordination. If you experience discomfort turning your head, look straight.

Again place your right leg at 90 degrees for this pose, four feet apart, heel to instep alignment. Turn the left foot slightly to the left. Square your hips forward. Inhale arms in T.

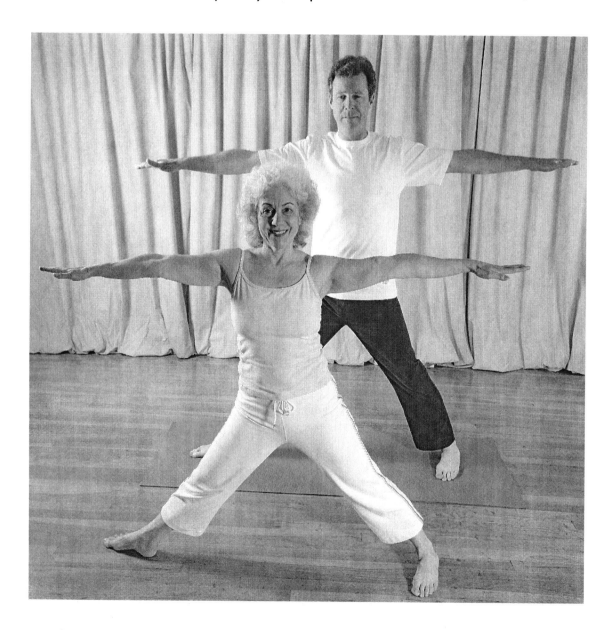

Exhale bend the right knee, look over the right knee. Tighten your left leg making it active, center your torso by bringing it back to center, make sure the knee is over the ankle and not beyond. Stay in this position for about three breaths.

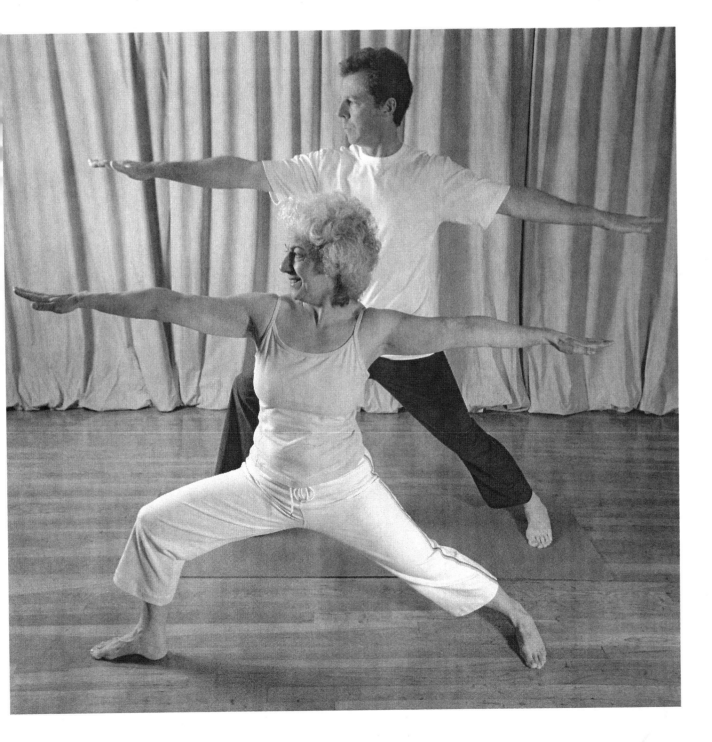

Coming out of Warrior II Pose
Straighten out your legs, bring your arms down by your side,
toes pointed forward.

Step your feet together.

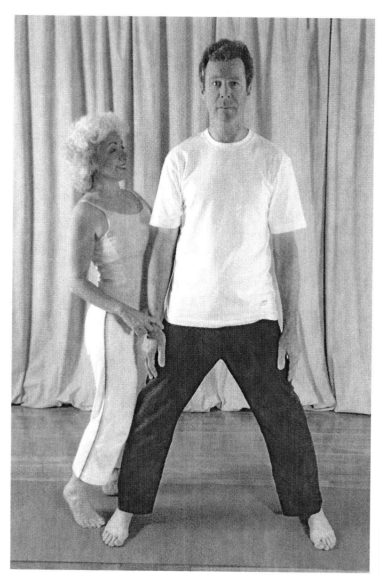 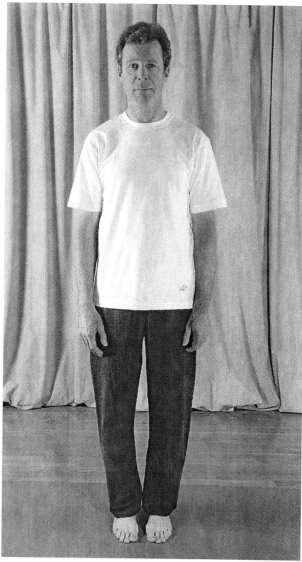

Repeat Warrior II on the other side.
Place your left leg at 90 degrees for this pose, four feet apart,
heel to instep alignment. Turn the right foot slightly to the right.
Square your hips forward. Inhale arms in T.

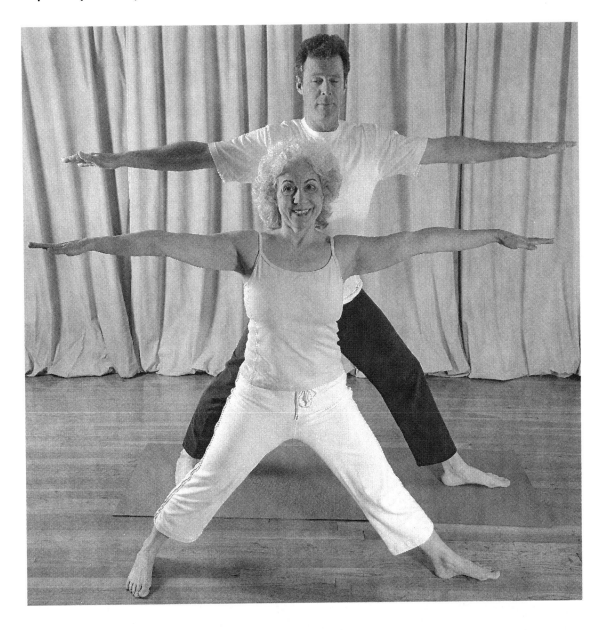

Exhale bend the left knee, look over the left knee. Tighten your right leg making it active, center your torso by bringing it back to center, make sure the knee is over the ankle and not beyond. Stay in this position for about three breaths.

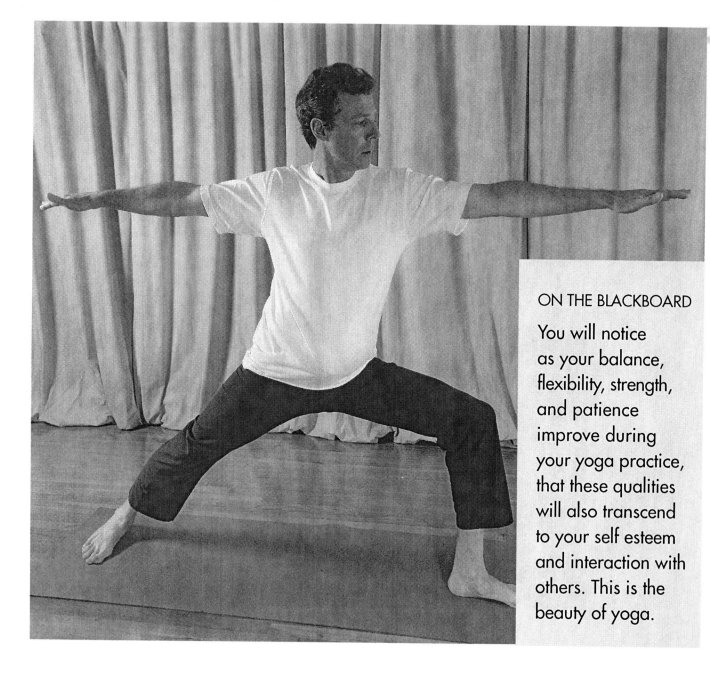

ON THE BLACKBOARD

You will notice as your balance, flexibility, strength, and patience improve during your yoga practice, that these qualities will also transcend to your self esteem and interaction with others. This is the beauty of yoga.

Coming out of Warrior II Pose
Straighten out your legs, bring your arms down by your side,
toes pointed forward.

Step your feet together.

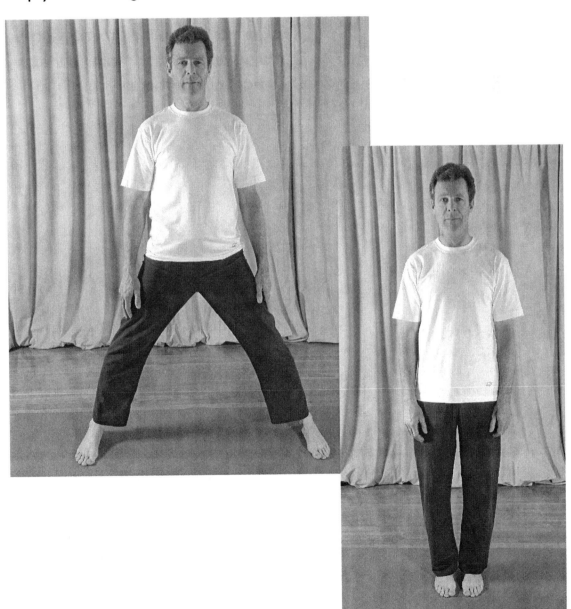

Knee Bend

This firms the quadriceps and buttocks. Do not attempt if you have knee pain.

Keep your legs together and lift your arms straight out in front of you with palms down. Rise up on the balls of your feet.

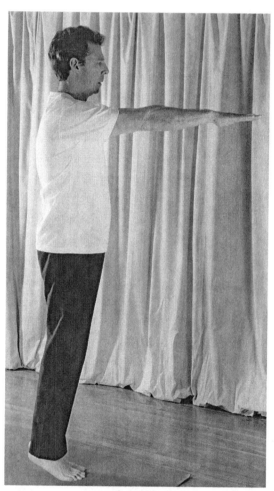

Exhale, bend your knees, and slowly lower yourself to the ground, finally resting on your back with your legs straight out in front of you.

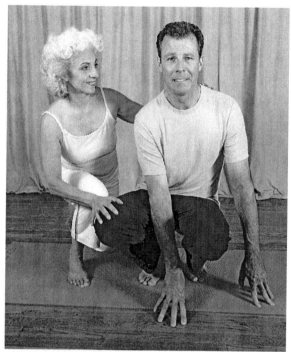

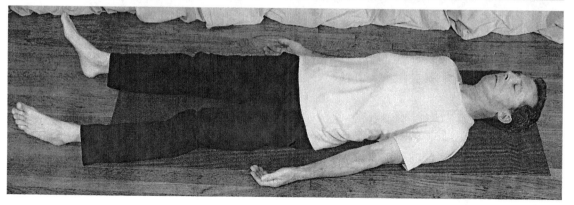

CHAPTER 7

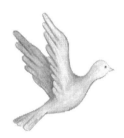

Relaxation

Corpse Pose

Walk your arms down, bringing shoulders away from your ears. Lift your chest slightly, tuck your shoulder blades under just a little, and relax. Roll your chin down to your chest, stretching the back of your neck. Make sure your legs are stretched to the width of the mat, your arms are just a few inches away from your body, your palms are up, and your eyes are closed.

Begin to slow down and quiet your breath. On every exhalation you will feel tension release from your body. Each time your mind wanders, acknowledge the thought and gently let it go, always returning back to the breath.

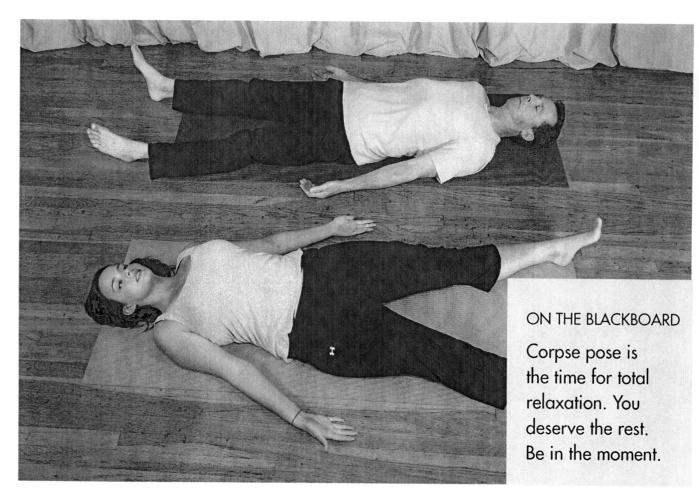

ON THE BLACKBOARD

Corpse pose is the time for total relaxation. You deserve the rest. Be in the moment.

Come out of Corpse by breathing in deeply. Wiggle your fingers and toes and gently move your head from side to side. Exhale. Breathe in deeply again and, with your arms overhead, take a good stretch. Breathe in deeply a third time and open your eyes.

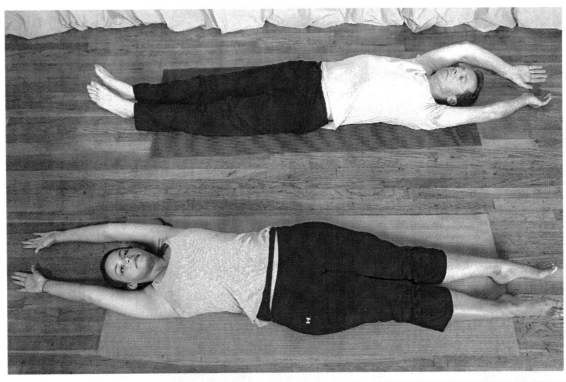

Bring your knees to your chest for Knee Hug Pose and rock from side to side several times in order to massage your spine.

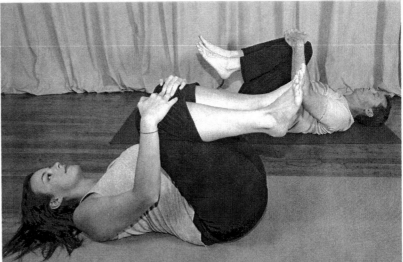

Roll onto your right side, curling into a fetal position. Remain here for a few more deep breaths.

Push yourself up by using your arms and not your back. Bring yourself into a comfortable seated position.

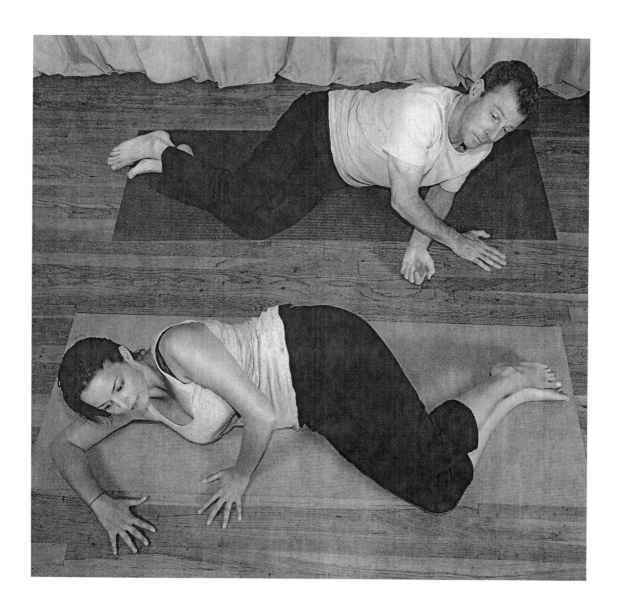

CHAPTER 8

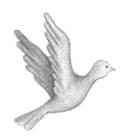

Meditation

Meditation

Sit in a comfortable position. Keep your spine erect and hands resting on your knees, thumb and index fingers touching, palms facing up or down. Eyes are closed. Keeping your eyes closed enables you to turn inward and not be distracted by outside stimuli. In order to clear the mind and stay focused, silently or out loud repeat a word such as love, peace, or om as you breathe slowly, deeply, and rhythmically. Stay in meditation for at least five minutes.

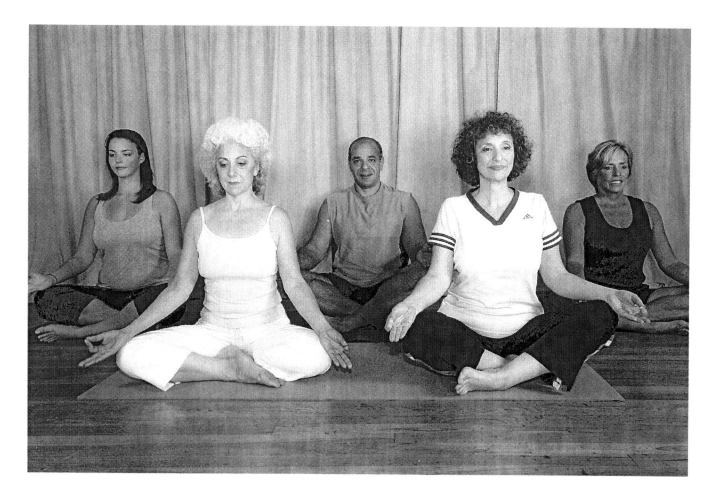

End of Session

Press your palms together in prayer by your heart and say, "Namaste," which means, I bow to the divine in you.

THANK YOU FOR JOINING US.
I hope this class inspired you to continue your journey.

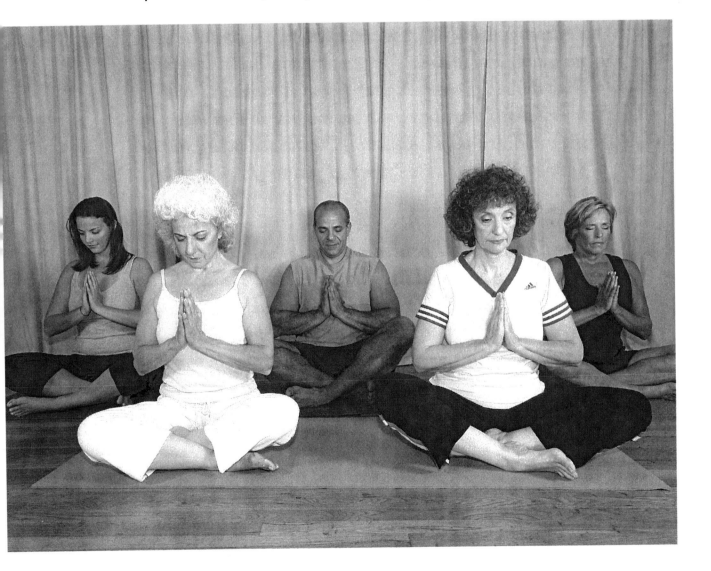

Hug a Tree

While attending classes at the Yoga Teacher's Training Institute we were given the option to hug a tree during the meditation walk. It wasn't mandatory; we could do it if we felt inspired to do so. I felt embarrassed and uncomfortable with this assignment. In fact, found it comical. I told myself that I wasn't going to participate in that aspect of the walk. As I began my walk, I reminded myself not to be so narrow-minded. Perhaps, I just might gain something from this experience.

The first tree that I noticed was beautiful. The trunk was perfectly rounded and its branches stretched gracefully up to the sky. It was the first time I really looked closely at a tree. However, I didn't feel the desire to hug it. I continued my walk looking for a tree that needed a hug. There it stood with its deformed trunk and branches. Not an attractive looking tree I thought. Who would hug this tree?

*Well, I reluctantly walked up to it, looked around hoping
no one was watching me hugging a tree. I slowly put my
arms around it, rested my head in the hollow part of the
trunk, and began to cry. I didn't want to let go. I felt
comforted by this seemingly imperfect work of nature.
I then realized that this tree didn't need me as much as
I needed it.*

*Consider doing this exercise, it may enhance your yoga
practice.*

CHAPTER 9

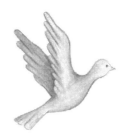

Questions

and

Answers

The purpose of the question and answer section is to provide you with a basic knowledge of yoga. For a deeper understanding of yoga's benefits and philosophy, please do further research. I recommend:

Dickman, Carol. BED TOP YOGA, and SEATED YOGA, DVD. Yoga Enterprises, Inc., 1999.

Budilovsky, J., Adamsom, E., THE COMPLETE IDIOT'S GUIDE TO MEDITATION. Alpha A. Pearson Education Company, Indiana, 2003.

Iyengar, B.K.S. LIGHT ON YOGA. Schoken Books. New York, 1966.

Stiles, M., STRUCTURAL YOGA THERAPY: ADAPTING TO THE INDIVIDUAL. Boston: Weiser Books, 2000.

I also enjoy the Yoga Journal and its website: www.yogajournal.com

What does the word yoga mean?
Yoga is a Sanskrit word meaning "to yoke" or "to unite." In a broader sense, to unite with your higher power. Sanskrit is a classical language of India.

What does uniting with your higher power have to do with yoga exercises?
Classical yoga is a path laid out by the Sage Patanjali more than 5,000 years ago. The path, which encompasses eight branches, or limbs, is a series of disciplines that purify the body and mind, preparing them to achieve enlightenment.

The Eight Limbs

1. Yamas—Nonviolence, truthfulness, moderation in all things, not stealing
2. Niyamas—Internal and external cleanliness, contentment, austerity, study of the sacred texts, awareness of the divine presence
3. Asanas—Postures
4. Pranayama—Control of the breath
5. Pratyahara—Withdrawal of the senses in order to still the mind
6. Dharana—Concentration
7. Dhyana—Meditation
8. Samadhi—A state of oneness with your higher power

Yoga asanas, which you just completed in this book, are only one part of the science and art of yoga. Because the Western cultures emphasize fitness, we mainly practice postures.

Are there other types of yoga?

Yes, some of the most popular are:

Iyengar Yoga—Developed by the yoga master B. K. S. Iyengar, this type of yoga emphasizes body alignment and the use of props such as blankets, blocks, and belts.

Bikram Yoga or Hot Yoga—This form is a series of yoga postures done in a room heated to about 95 degrees Fahrenheit.

Ashtanga Yoga—This set of poses is performed in the same order every time and is practiced very fast.

Kundalini Yoga—A spiritual type of yoga, this focuses not only on asanas but on breathing, meditation, and chanting.

Hatha Yoga—It emphasizes postures, breathing techniques, and meditation.

Is yoga a religion?
Yoga is not a religion, however it will enhance your spirituality.

Why practice the yoga postures in bare feet?
You want to connect with the earth and feel grounded. Yoga postures allow the feet to stretch and breathe. Feet that are stretched provide a firm foundation for standing postures. Also, bare feet prevent slipping.

What is the purpose of a yoga mat?
A yoga or sticky mat not only prevents slipping but is considered your own spiritual place.

Why is breathing an important part of yoga?
You want to fill the body with oxygen and prana. Prana is energy. In Chinese it is called chi and in Japanese, ki. Most of us don't breathe correctly. We breathe with our chest, creating short and shallow breaths. As a result, our bodies

are starving for oxygen. Natural breathing is from the abdominal area. It is slow, deep, and rhythmical. As you inhale your stomach rises, and as you exhale the stomach falls. The chest moves only slightly. We were born to breathe this way.

Why did our breathing shift from the abdomen to the chest?
As we grow older, we take breathing for granted and forget to breathe properly. We develop poor breathing habits.

How do yoga postures help to maintain good posture?
They help by stretching, elongating, and aligning the spine. Movement of the spine is necessary for the health of discs and joints. Aging, injuries, and bad habits result in poor posture.

What are some of the health benefits of yoga?
With frequent practice, yoga benefits the whole person with increased flexibility, strength, range of motion, and blood circulation; better breathing; mental calmness; reduced stress; and greater body awareness.

What is meditation?
Meditation clears the mind and connects you with your higher power. Your mind likes to chitchat. It likes to think of all kinds of things. This continuous chitchat clutters the mind with too much stuff, stuff that makes it difficult to think clearly, make decisions, and stay calm. With a clear mind, you won't become frazzled so easily.

Meditation gives the mind something constructive to do. You tell your mind to focus on one thing: your breath, a repeated word such as love or peace, or a repeated sound—om, for example. Meditation also takes you within yourself and helps you to connect with your higher power. Be patient! Meditation takes practice.

Why repeat the sound of om during meditation?
It is thought that om is the sound the universe makes. Chant it in three syllables: ah-ooh-mmm. Ahoohmmm. Say these sounds as you exhale. Make them musical. Can you feel the vibration? You can chant it out loud or to yourself.

What is the meaning of Namaste?
At the beginning or at the end of a yoga session, say the word Namaste, pronounced nah-mas-day. It is a Sanskrit word that means "I bow to the divine in you" or "the light in me bows to the light in you."

Where you can find:
IT'S TIME FOR YOGA, ROLL OUT THE MAT

Copies of this book may be purchased through
AuthorHouse.com, BarnesAndNoble.com, Borders.com.,
Amazon.com.

You can also obtain a copy by ordering it from your favorite
book store.

For more information regarding Diana Dantuono and
her book, please visit the author's website at
www.itstimeforyoga.com or email her at
diana@itstimeforyoga.com

A portion of the proceeds will be donated to Vitamin Angels to
eliminate Vitamin A deficient childhood blindness.

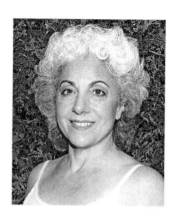

ABOUT THE AUTHOR

Diana Dantuono is a registered yoga instructor who has practiced and taught yoga since 2000. She teaches on Long Island, New York, and has conducted workshops on the philosophy and benefits of yoga. She has been involved in yoga projects for the mentally ill and for cancer survivors.

Diana holds a certificate of advanced study in educational administration from Hofstra University, a master's in special education from Long Island University, a post-baccalaureate certificate in gerontology from Adelphi University, and is certified in English as a Second Language teacher. She also holds a certificate in Reiki, Level II.

When she is not practicing or teaching yoga, Diana is a special education teacher for the New York State Office of Mental Health.